How to Stay Young and Fit No Matter How Old You Get

Anti-Aging Secrets

Sharon J. Scott

Copyright

Contents

Introduction

We age because we must not because we want to. Getting older is not on anybody's list of things to do but it happens to us all. The question is what can we do to stay younger, longer?

Turn on the TV, pick up a magazine or walk into any drug store and you will be bombarded with products designed to make you look younger. Plastic surgeons offer to trim, tuck and lift so that you look younger and people pay. The quest for youth is indeed a big money maker but who really benefits?

Do expensive creams and lotions really ward off aging? Can a doctor perform miracles with a scalpel? Yes and no. There is no easy answer to that, because some of the ingredients in the lotions and creams can help some and some plastic surgery can have attractive results that make you look younger. However, for many, these are expensive and impractical solutions.

Plastic surgery carries a high degree of risk and you often end up looking worse than you did before surgery. Wrinkles look better than overly tightened skin that has pulled your eyebrows up in a look of constant surprise. The problem with our quest for youth is that we focus too much on the exterior.

We want to look young, but why just in looks. Why should we not feel young and think young at the same time as looking young. It is possible and this book will tell you how.

Aging affects our brains and our bodies, both inside and out. If you want to tackle aging, you need to take a whole body approach to staying young. Wrinkle creams do not help you feel young nor do they help your body work better, just as it did when you were younger.

The secret to youth is that you work on your mind and body at the same time. Youthfulness begins from the inside out.

What is the Aging Process?

The minute we are born, we begin to age. Aging is a predetermined process that is programed into our cells. Our DNA is a blueprint of ourselves, and it has the instructions for aging in its helix. We age because our genes tell us too. This is why some people begin to show signs of aging before others.

As we age, we experience degenerative changes to our organs, tissues, bones and our skin. Telemeres are parts of our DNA, located at the ends of our chromosomes. When a cell divides, the telomere shortens; aging the cell and eventually, the cell dies. What happens to us on a cellular level translates what happens to us as a whole, we age and we die.

We cannot stop the aging process, but we can control some factors that influence it. In order to slow down the aging process, we need to understand it first.

Knowing how your body is changing helps you learn how to slow down the aging process, keeping you younger and healthier for longer.

Cardiovascular System

Aging slows down the heart rate and the heart itself will often enlarge. Arteries and blood vessels, especially those in the heart, stiffen so your heart is forced to work harder. This contributes to high blood pressure and a whole host of age related cardiac problems.

Muscles, Bones, and Joints

Bones lose density and they shrink slightly. As we age, we shorten slightly. Shrinking bones and a loss of bones density increase the probability of breaks and fractures as the bones become brittle. Muscle flexibility declines as does muscle strength causing overall weakness and balance issues. Coordination begins to decline. Joints lose their natural lubrication as cartilage wears down, causing arthritis and inflammation.

Digestive System

Constipation is a common problem as the digestive system begins to slow. Medications can contribute to this, as well as not being hydrated enough, not being active enough or not getting a proper diet. As we age, those are all common factors and it can affect the digestive system.

Urinary Tract

Weakened muscles in the pelvic floor can cause urinary incontinence and partial to full loss of bladder control can happen. For men, as their prostrate enlarges with age, it causes incontinence as well and for women, menopause has the same effect. Kidneys no longer work as efficiently, allowing toxins to build up in the blood.

Memory

As we age, we start to lose our memory. Although some age related illnesses greatly affect the memory, it is normal to begin to lose our memory as we age. Remembering new things becomes difficult and even trying to come of words that we know can be challenging.

Ears and Eyes

Our vision weakens with age and cataracts are common. Focus becomes harder, especially up close and the glare from lights can be more bothersome as you age. We lose our ability to hear higher frequencies and indeed, our hearing as a whole begins to decline.

Skin

Our skin loses its elasticity so it sags and is more fragile. The skin itself is thinner and bruises form easily. We produce less natural oil as we age so it makes our skin drier and skin tags, age spots and wrinkles form.

Teeth

Dry mouth is a side effect of many common medications, especially for high blood pressure and this contributes to gum disease. Gums begin to recede, and infection and decay of the mouth becomes more common.

The above are the basics of how aging takes a toll on the body. Knowing how aging targets the body allows us to fight back, warding off the major signs of aging while keeping our body and mind healthy.

Wellness and Anti-Aging

In order to stay young, you need to be well. Wellness and health is not the same thing, although they are related.

In order to stay young and to fight aging, you need to be well and that means that your wellness is a factor. Health is your bodily health, and that is what you are your doctor work together on; keeping your weight healthy, ensuring that your blood pressure is okay, that you are disease free and feeling good.

Wellness is a broader term and your health is included in wellness. Wellness is your overall health, your fitness, and how your mind and spirit are. Wellness is how your mind, body and spirit are and to stay young, your wellness matters.

Your body, mind and spirit are all connected and so if one is lacking, then it will affect everything. If your mental health is not healthy, your body and spirit is not healthy. If one is ailing, the others are going to be unwell as well.

Doctors tell us to be fit; we see fitness and health information all over but having a healthy body is only a piece of the puzzle. Your health is something that can be measured but your wellness is more subjective.

In other words, only you can diagnose the state of your own wellness. You can test your fitness level at the gym but your wellness level has no such test.

To help keep yourself young, you need to be well, not just healthy and fit. Your wellness matters and since you are the only one who can judge how well you really are, you need to start paying attention.

Your life is a balance of body, mind and spirit and when they are all balanced, you are well. When they are not balanced, you are unwell.

Because aging affects your mind and body, your wellness helps you stay young because it can help ward off the signs of aging.

Being well is not only good for you in terms of feeling young, but it boosts your health and it boosts your spirits. Being well means that you are happy and who does not want more happiness in their life? Sadly, many people go through life experiencing very little happiness and that is why they are unwell.

As you age, your body is under stress. Stress can cause your mental state to become agitated or even depressed and that in turn affects your spiritual state.

Learning how to keep that balance will help your body be able to resist the stress of aging, and it can help slow down that march of time that so many people dread. The secret to anti-aging is not found in a bottle or via surgery; the secret is that you hold the power of anti-aging already. You just have to learn how to use it.

Your diet, your fitness level and your lifestyle habits all contribute to your wellness. You can eat well, but if your only exercise is to go from the couch to the kitchen and back again, you cannot claim to have a high wellness factor.

If you eat well and work out often but you smoke, drink and are living with chronic stress, you are also unwell. In order to be well, you need to examine your entire lifestyle, your nutritional intake, your health, your fitness level, your mental health and your overall spiritual wellbeing.

If you are constantly going from crisis to crisis in your life, that ages you even faster! Unless you have balance in your life, your aging will be accelerated and that is the opposite of what you want to happen.

The best way to stop the process of aging in its tracks is by focusing on your wellness. Several companies out there want you to believe that they hold the secret to anti-aging in their formulas. If you drink this or take that supplement, the hands of time will reverse; or so they say.

Companies want to make money on people looking for an easy out for beating the aging process. There is no easy out, if you are not willing to make the changes that you need to make to look and feel younger, then this book is not for you.

For those of you willing to put in the effort instead of trying to buy your youth back, this book will help. You will learn how to increase your wellness by increasing your fitness, your health and your mental and spiritual state.

To keep the signs of aging at bay, you need to be fit mentally and physically. Does that mean you have to live in a gym to stay young? Not at all!

You might be surprised at how easy it is to help stay young by staying active. Learning to engage your mind while staying fit and healthy all contribute to your wellness factor, which keeps you young.

Once you begin to start to follow the directions in this book, you will notice a difference. You will begin to feel better, and when your body begins to feel better, you start to feel better.

Remember, our goal is to not just help you look younger, but to feel younger and better. Products sold in stores are targeted to your exterior, they help with wrinkles and fine lines, but they do not target the inside changes.

This full body approach is the best way to not only improve your mental and physical health, but it will make you look and feel younger!

Stop the signs of aging in their tracks by giving your body what it needs to stay healthy and the signs of aging will start to diminish. Stop looking in the mirror and seeing somebody old; see the new, younger you thanks to this book.

It is important to note that you cannot pick and choose what parts of this book to follow. The entire point of this chapter is to teach you how wellness is a multi-faceted concept. Wellness is a combination of many factors and if you let even one factor slide, your wellness factor slides as well. To stay young, you need to stay well.

Staying Spiritually Young

Everybody has heard the phrase that you are only as old as you feel but few really understand it. Feeling young spiritually helps you stay young physically. If you decide that you are old, then you feel old.

Your spiritual health is one part of many that helps you to stay young and youthful. Most people know how to work on their mental health, they do puzzles or other things to keep their brain occupied and they know to exercise to stay physically fit but how do you stay spiritually fit?

Getting older does not mean that you have to have dinner by before five pm and in bed by eight pm. Getting older does not mean that you have to give up on the ideals and pleasures that you had when you were younger.

The minute that you do give up on those ideals and pleasures and the minute that you start going doing the things that "old people do" is the minute that you start to get old. You cannot turn back the clock on how old you are but you are fully in control of how old you feel!

Does that mean that you have to learn the current slang being used by the youth of today and adopt their fashion trends? No, it just means that you do what makes you feel happy. If it makes you happy to wear a hat, then wear a hat! If you want to take up yoga, take up yoga.

Do not let anybody tell you that you are "too old" or worry that you might be judged. If you want to learn how to do something because you have a desire to learn, then do it.

In fact, doing new things is one of the best ways to stay spiritually young. In your youth, you were constantly having new experiences and learning new things but as we age, we tend to fall into a rut.

Life becomes predictable and even boring. You do not have to live a boring life just because you are getting older. If you want to feel young, recapture the spirit of youth by trying new things! Try a cuisine you have not tried before, visit some place new, learn a new language, or try a new hobby.

Why stop exploring the world just because you are getting older? Make a habit of doing and learning new things so that you are constantly on a path of discovery. Join clubs, volunteer, take classes and fill in the empty hours with things that make you happy.

When we are younger, nothing makes us feel young like spending time with our friends or making new friends so always be open to meeting new people and going out. The opportunities in the prior sentence will allow you to expand your social horizons, helping you to feel happy and content.

You do not have to limit your friendships only to people your own age either. Keep an open mind about people and you will find that it is easy to connect to people of all ages.

Having friends that are both older and younger than you are helps you keep a fresh perspective on the world. There are no rules that say that you have to only be friends with your age group. Talking about the past is one thing, but those good old days are just memories.

When you live in the past, you tend to let the present go by without noticing. That is not healthy for you spiritually.

When you feel useful, you feel spiritually fulfilled. Feeling useless is a sure fire way to feel old so never let yourself feel useless.

Do things that make you happy, get out of the house and find positive ways to make yourself feel useful. Volunteering was mentioned earlier, it is a great way to help others. Helping others helps boost your self-esteem, your feeling of self-worth, and it is spiritually fulfilling.

A happy person is a young person. Aging is not fun and it can be hard to keep a good outlook; it is easy to get into the habit of worrying. That is a habit that needs to be broken though because a healthy spirit helps make you stay healthy in body.

Worrying less means that your immune system works better and all of the problems that come with age will seem less overwhelming.

Do the things that make you happy. Even simple things can help restore a happy mental state. When you give up being happy, you end up giving up on really living and then your spiritual health declines quickly. Remember, that in order to be well, you have to also be well spiritually.

Feed your spiritual side by not letting age define you, staying active, do things that you enjoy, stay useful and be social. Feeling younger helps you be younger.

Adjust Your Attitude

Your attitude is a reflection of how you see the world. If you see the world in a negative way, you will have a negative attitude.

If you see the world in a positive way, you will have a positive attitude. You probably do not need us to tell you that one of the secrets to staying young is to have a good attitude but we are going to tell you anyways. One of the secrets to staying young is to have a good attitude.

Your attitude is shaped by your perceptions. You can say that your attitude is a culmination of your experience during your lifetime. Bad things happen sometimes but you do not have to have a bad attitude, which is up to you.

Your personality and your attitude are closely intertwined. What does this have to do with staying young? Quite a bit, actually.

A negative attitude leads to a negative personality, which is unhealthy. Negativity robs you of your ability to enjoy your life.

Enjoying life is one of the secrets to staying young so your attitude is most certainly very important in your ability to stay young. Negative attitudes contribute to making you age faster and it is detrimental to your health. You have every reason to adjust your attitude because it helps you to stay young.

Naturally, it is not possible to just close your eyes and adjust your attitude, if it were only that simple. Changing your attitude takes a lot of work but if you want to stay young, it is worth it because you will find that life is so much happier and easier to deal with when your attitude is healthy and positive!

Your outlook on life is not set in stone; you can change it, as long as you want to. Wanting to change is a key theme in this book; this book promises to help you look and feel younger but only if you put in the effort to follow our directions.

Only you can gauge what your attitude is like. This requires you to be brutally honest with yourself. How do you view the world? How do you view your life? Are you happy?

What aspects of your life are you not happy with? What bothers you the most and more importantly can you change it? If you can change it, begin to change it! If you cannot change it, let it go.

Quite often, the past holds us trapped. When mistakes from our past or regrets that we have their grip on us, we find it hard to move on.

Moving on is necessary in order to reclaim a positive outlook. Bitterness and anger are just as toxic as taking poison. When you take poison, it starts to shut your body down, harming you. Bitterness and anger are toxic emotions, harming your mental and spiritual health, which contributes to premature aging.

Your negative outlook and attitude can be making you age faster than you should be. They take root inside your head and they taint everything that you see or do. Because one person hurt you years ago, you might be suspicious of all people.

Going through life trusting nobody and carrying anger and resentment around is a terrible burden and it is a burden that many people choose to carry.

Letting go is not easy. Letting go does not mean that you have forgotten what has hurt you, it means that you have learned from it and you will not let it happen again so there is no reason to carry it around with you. If you have anything in your past that you are still holding tight to; anything negative, let it go.

What are the benefits of letting go compared to the benefits of holding on? When you make a list and see them in black and white, letting go of the hurtful things in your past make sense.

You have a choice to reclaim your happiness by letting go; recognizing this choice is the first step. Until now, you may not have realized that you could let go because you have carried the hurt for so long.

Every negative experience is a learning experience. What did you learn from it? What could you have done differently and what signs did you miss that could have prevented the situation from happening in the first place?

Once you sit and analyze it, you can recognize that you will not let it happen again because you have learned and you can simply let go. That means that you have to forgive the other person.

What was done was done and every minute that you spend thinking about the past is time that you are taking away from your future and your present. When you start to think about the past, make a conscious effort to focus on the present.

Stop letting yourself dwell on the past and you will slowly but surely stop reliving painful memories and start focusing on creating positive memories and experiences instead.

It helps to remember that we cannot control everything that happens in life. We cannot control other people or external events; we can only control our reactions to these things.

If somebody is mean to you, it is not a reflection of you; it is a reflection of them. Stop taking things personally and if you cannot control it, let it go. Worrying about things that you have zero control over is a big reason why your personality can be negative. Worry is just another toxic emotion and one that you need to get rid of.

Do you have anything to gain from not being positive? No, you have more to lose by being negative than you have to gain from being positive.

Being positive is a boost to your mental and physical health and it helps keep your body healthy. Stress takes a serious toll on the body and when you are fighting the signs of aging, the last thing you want to do is add additional stress to your body.

Adjusting your attitude means that you are helping your body be healthy, it keeps you mentally fit and better yet, it keeps you spiritually fit. If you want to be well, then you need to be positive.

Start finding more reasons to adjust your attitude for the better and you will find that you will start to feel better about yourself and about life in general. Your attitude can mean that you enjoy life or go through it grumpy but a bad outlook is no way to live and it will age you just as quickly as physical stress will.

When you start to think or say something negative, simply stop yourself and replace it with something positive. If what you were about to say had no value other than to be negative, then it does not need to be said.

The more you weed out your negative thoughts by replacing them with positive thoughts, the less negative thoughts you will have.

It is a slow process but it will turn your negative mindset into a positive one, one that will help you feel better. Feeling better helps you look and feel younger.

Emotional Health

Your emotional health helps you stay young as well. Negative emotions lead to a negative attitude and from the prior chapter, a negative attitude is a surefire way to age you even faster.

Your emotional health matters and as you age, it can be harder to keep your emotions healthy and positive. However, that is all the more reason for why you need to keep your emotional health monitored.

Staying emotionally healthy is a challenge for anybody, no matter what their age is, but when we are aging, that is when it becomes harder. Neglecting your emotional health is simply not healthy and so many people neglect it.

Emotional health, when it is low, causes bodily harm and mental harm. Low emotional health can lead to depression and stress related illnesses. Neither of which will allow you to look or feel young.

Take control of your emotional health today. Take a good look at the people around you. Are you surrounded by people who lift you up or by people who encourage you to be miserable?

Negative people love to spread their negativity and if you have a negative friend or acquaintance, it will take a toll on your emotional health.

Limit your time with people who do not support you and make you happy. If you cannot cut all contact with them, limit your interactions the best you can, while still being polite.

Remember, in the prior chapter it was mentioned that you cannot control other people; just your own reactions so if somebody is negative, reply positively and then walk away.

If they frown, smile and go about your business. You do not gain anything by matching their negative state and the more time you spend around them, the harder it becomes to stay emotionally healthy.

You know the type of people that are not good to be around; the people who never take personal responsibility, the people who do nothing but complain, and the people who never say anything positive about anybody or any situation.

If any of the above describes you, then you have something else to work on. Does complaining ever do any good? No. If something is bothering you, do something about it or let it go.

Ever had a meal with a chronic complainer? They get their food; complain to the waiter, get their food back and it is acceptable this time but they spend the entire meal complaining about the mistake.

That is not an emotionally healthy person because there is no benefit to complaining about something that is no longer relevant.

These are the habits that you need to break and if you know people like this, you need to stay away. Protect your own emotional health by adopting healthy emotional habits.

One habit that you need to break is the habit of feeling guilty. People love to place blame on anybody but themselves and eventually, somebody will point the finger at you. You know that it is not your fault so do not ever accept blame that other people are putting on you.

Accepting or allowing blame into your life will only bring you stress and negative emotions. If somebody is trying to place undue blame on you that is somebody that you need to break contact with.

Another thing is that you need to be careful to not allow them to engage you in an argument. When they get your emotions running high and you go on the defensive, they have won.

You will be in a negative mindset, your emotions will be all over the place and you will have gained nothing. When somebody tries to force their guilt on you, do not let them but do not argue. Walk away.

Bottling in your emotions is unhealthy as well. Staying strong does not mean that you never cry or that things do not bother you. Having a good cry does not make you weak and it can actually help you feel better.

Crying can be a way to relief bottled up emotional stress. Crying all the time, however, is not healthy. Constant crying goes with constant complaining; neither of them accomplishes anything positive and should be avoided.

If you need to cry, cry. Crying helps release that pent up feeling of sorrow, anger and hurt. Forcing yourself to not cry means you hold those emotions inside yourself and those emotions are toxic.

You will suffer if you hold onto those for very long because it will start to affect your mood, your personality and your mindset in very negative ways and you will become one of those people that you were just warned to steer clear of.

Laughter is good for the soul and it is good for the body. Laughter helps fight stress and it helps to fight negative emotions. When you laugh, your body releases endorphins; endorphins help make you feel good.

Laughing is great for erasing pain, clearing away stress and chasing away the blues. Laughing boosts the immune system and it provides exercise for your heart muscles.

When you feel that your emotional health is out of balance, find something to laugh about. Put on your favorite comedy, talk to a friend and reminisce about funny memories that you share or just act silly. Laughter is the best way to lighten your soul and make yourself feel young again.

Staying Stress Free

Stress accelerates the aging process. The telomeres, the part of the chromosomes that becomes smaller as we age are affected by stress. Chronic stress makes us age faster than we already are.

If you want to stay young, then you need to stay stress free or stress will cause problems with your health and it will age you. When you are stressed, your body produces cortisol, which is not intended to be in the body for a long period of time.

Chronic stress means that your body has a constant supply of cortisol in it, and cortisol causes the telomeres in your chromosomes to shorten, which causes the cells to age faster.

In addition to affecting the telomeres, stress also causes other problems in the body such as weight gain, insomnia, suppressed immune system, digestive problems and problems with the central nervous system.

Stress causes our bodies to go into fight or flight mode thanks to the cortisol that is released. Cortisol triggers changes in our bodies that are supposed to help us get through the stressful situation but when the stress remains, cortisol remains in our bodies, causing damage.

Alzheimer's is a terrible disease and chronic stress has been linked to earlier onset of the disease.

Females are even more prone to developing Alzheimer's if they are under chronic stress. Even if somebody does not develop Alzheimer's chronic stress hastens the brain's aging process, causing memory loss and leading to somebody being confused easier. Your brain will stay younger if you stay stress free.

Another hormone that stress causes our body to produce is adrenaline, which can cause loss of hearing, loss of vision, increased blood pressure and a faster heart rate. Chronic stress keeps the adrenaline levels in the body higher than they should be and that will cause a decrease in vision and hearing.

Stress itself causes damage, but the mere thought of stress or even anticipating stress also causes our cells to age faster. If somebody is already experiencing chronic stress, the anticipation of an upcoming stressful event causes even greater cellular aging.

Just thinking about being stressed can age you; a perfect reason for why if you want to stay younger for longer, you need to manage your stress levels.

When you are stressed, insomnia is often a side effect. However, when you do not get enough sleep that also accelerates the aging process. Getting enough sleep is important not only for your health, but for your stress levels as well. Your body knows how much sleep it needs, but most people need between six to eight hours of sleep. Not enough sleep makes it harder for you to function and it can impair your brain function.

To get enough sleep, limit your computer and TV watching so that you have them turned off two hours before going to bed. The artificial light from your TV and computer screens can actually disrupt your sleep cycle, making it harder for you to fall asleep.

Getting light exercise during the day will help as well and limit your caffeine intake to mornings only, nothing in the late afternoon or evening.

Daily meditation is a great way to help keep your stress away. Meditation is soothing, easy and anybody can do it. A five to ten minute meditation session will help you feel more centered, less anxious and less stressed.

Meditation morning and night is a good way to begin and end your day with a clear mind and a rested spirit. Some people prefer to use guided meditations, where somebody is walking them through the meditation process.

Guided meditations can be found on YouTube or other places on line or they can be downloaded onto phones, tablets, and other media devices for you to listen to.

Doing your own meditation is easy as well. Meditation nearly always begins with deep breathing exercises. Deep breathing exercises are helpful for calming stress and anxiety because you start to feel better almost immediately. The increase of oxygen in your body due to deep breathing exercises is rejuvenating to both body and mind. You can do them anywhere, at any time to calm yourself down and keep stress from building up.

Sit straight up and take a deep breathe in, starting with your belly and feel your stomach expand with air. Imagine that as you inhale that the air begins to fill your stomach first, and then your chest will expand. If your chest expands before your stomach, you are breathing wrong.

It might be helpful to place one hand on your stomach so you can feel your stomach rise as you begin to inhale. Do not inhale quickly, but rather take in a long, slow breath and then hold it for a few seconds and then exhale it very slowly, out your mouth.

Repeat two to three times for a quick stress relief and do this for a few minutes for a nice, simple meditation exercise.

Take time for yourself. If you are always at somebody else's beck and call, when do you have time for yourself?

Do things that you love to do and do them daily so you can balance out the stress that you encounter daily with something that you love to do. Hobbies are great for relieving tension.

Learn to say no and do not feel guilty about doing so. You need to set boundaries and enforce them or else you will be in a constant battle with other people who are trying to test your boundaries.

Say no and mean it and the energy vampires in your life will fade away for good, helping you have a happier and stress-free existence.

Take up yoga or even tai chi. Both of these are great for helping to keep the body flexible, help keep you fit and healthy and they incorporate mind relaxation techniques that help you shed the stress while feeling good.

Yoga and tai chi are calming, relaxing and therapeutic. Look for local classes near you. Sign up, it will do your body and mind good.

A cluttered environment has been proven to be stressful; even if you do not realize it, it is. When you have to search and search to find something that is stressful.

Organize yourself so that everything has a place. Not only will your place look clean, but also you will find that you do not feel as overwhelmed as you used to. It is a simple trick for helping making small changes to help you feel less stressed.

When you can manage your stress, you can help prevent premature aging. The longer you are operating with chronic stress, the faster you will age. Stress relieving techniques are necessary if you want to be and feel healthier and younger.

Eat to Stay Young

Good nutrition is the foundation for keeping your brain and your body healthy. Not only will proper nutrition keep you healthy, but also it will keep you young.

Every store sells supplements that are designed to improve memory, help your body work well and to help you feel younger but they are not a substitute for eating well. Unless you are giving your body what it needs to be healthy, it will have problems fighting off the signs and troubles that come with aging.

Just like we need to have proper nutrition for our bodies to develop properly, proper nutrition is necessary to keep everything working properly. When we stop eating right, we suffer the consequences of it, usually through various illnesses or health complaints.

Eating right will also help us ward off things that tend to age us, such as free radicals and other toxins that end up in our bodies. Good nutrition is a proactive way to help yourself stay and feel young.

We require a certain minimum amount of minerals, vitamins and food daily in order to keep our bodies and brains functioning at their best. Staying young means that you not only meet or exceed these limits but you also ensure that you eat foods rich in antioxidants. Just by adding the right foods to your diet, you can help fight the signs of aging, from the inside out.

You see plenty of fad diets that promise you excellent health and eternal youth, but many fad diets are not healthy. They focus on one area of nutrition but not the others.

The only way to stay healthy is to eat well; three main meals a day and snacks in between. Eating between meals helps keep your blood sugar levels stable and it will help keep you from overeating during mealtime as well.

The problem with the wrong types of foods is that they are so readily available and cheap. Fast foods and processed food generally make up at least 75% of the average person's diet and that is not healthy. Processed foods are full of sugar, artificial ingredients, preservatives and other unhealthy ingredients.

You are getting food, but it is far from being nutritious. Processing removes most of the nutrients from the food and the addition of artificial ingredients makes processed food an all-around bad choice in terms of your health.

If you want to stay younger, skip processed foods especially those with trans fats, processed sugars and artificial ingredients and preservatives. The abundance of convenient food products that are cheap but far from healthy is responsible for a health crisis, one of malnutrition and obesity.

Artificial ingredients make your body work harder to process them and some of them are even dangerous, especially artificial sweeteners.

If you want to eat to stay healthy, start eating fresh. Skip packaged food and go for the fresh. Eat organic as much as possible because organic food does not contain fertilizers and pesticides that other produce contains.

Many people think that if they simply rinse off their fruits and vegetables that they are able to wash off all of the residue left behind by commercial fertilizers and pesticides but that is not true. Because they wash into the soil, they are actually drawn up into the produce so you are ingesting small amounts, to avoid this, buy organic.

White rice and white flour can cause digestive issues. Switch to whole grains and you will find that you have less digestive problems.

Start reading food labels and if something contains high fructose corn syrup or anything that is hydrogenated or partially hydrogenated do not buy it. Processed foods are rich with these unhealthy ingredients so just leave them on the shelf, where they belong.

If more people stopped buying these unhealthy foods, they would no longer be so cheap and readily available. They remain popular because there is a high demand for them but change starts with you. Your health matters and if you want to look and feel younger, what you put into your body should matter too.

Dehydration is a major problem for many people and they do not even know it. Without enough water, our cells cannot move needed nutrients in and toxins out. Without water, we die.

We can live without food for longer than we can without water. Many people do not get enough water daily and are in a constant state of mild dehydration, which causes them to look older than they are.

Healthy skin is hydrated skin and no amount of moisturizer can make up for the fact that somebody is not drinking enough water. The problem is that too many people think that any beverage will replace water.

Coffee and tea is made with water, so it must be the same or even soda but this type of thinking is not only wrong, it is unhealthy. Although it will help to hydrate the body to some degree, there is no substitute for water.

The recommended amount of water to drink daily is six to eight glasses of water daily. If you want your skin to look plump and smooth, you need to have water. Dehydration causes wrinkles to form and the skin to appear dull and sallow.

Water keeps your body functioning smoothly and keeps your skin hydrated and healthy; giving you that youthful appearance you want.

Changing from a mostly processed diet to a fresh diet can be hard for some, but really, cooking at home saves you money in the long run over buying fast food or processed food.

Instead of buying frozen, ready to heat meals, make your own meals ahead of time and freeze them yourself. The amount of flavor that you get from fresh food over processed is amazing.

Processed food is often lacking flavor and texture so that is why they are filled with fillers and artificial ingredients; they are trying to fool you into thinking that it is healthy and tasty but it is not healthy for your body or your waistline. Not only is cooking and fixing your own meals tasty and healthy, but it gives you something to do.

Staying active is important if you want to look and feel young and many find that cooking is something that they enjoy. Meals do not have to be complicated to be flavorful.

Add more fish to your diet. Trans-fats are bad fat but not all fat is bad for you. Fish contains the good type of fat, Omega-3 fatty acids. We need these good fats to help our cardiovascular health, our mental health and our overall health.

Omega-3 fatty acids are antioxidants, so when you eat them, they enter the body to attack toxins and elements in our bodies that cause us to get sick or that weakens our cells. Many of the toxins that cause our cells to age prematurely can be shed by eating antioxidants, such as Omega-3 fatty acids.

Omega-3 fatty acids are also anti-inflammatory, and because joint inflammation is common with older people, eating tuna and salmon is a natural way to get relief. Omega-3 fatty acid also helps the skin stay firm and elastic, keeping it from getting dry. If you do not like to eat fish, take fish oil supplements daily.

Whole grains are not only a good source of fiber, but they help you feel full, help keep your blood sugar stable and they are a good source of healthy carbohydrate energy.

A diet including whole grains is a healthy diet; helping to combat stroke, high blood pressure, diabetes, breast cancer, colon cancer, and heart disease.

Swap out flour tortillas and white bread for whole-wheat tortillas and whole grain wheat bread. Switch to whole grain cereal and pasta for delicious meals that help you feel better. Oats, brown rice, barley and faro are also good whole grain choices that will help keep your digestive system healthy and regular and your body feeling good.

Not all vegetables are created equal and for many people, green vegetables are not their favorite. However, cruciferous vegetables are a powerhouse of nutrition and should become part of your daily diet. They contain sulfur, which is necessary to keeping your skin looking healthy and it provides energy.

They are antioxidants so they help rid your body of toxins and cancer causing agents, all of which help age you. What are cruciferous vegetables?

Brussels sprouts, kale, cauliflower, cabbage and broccoli are all cruciferous vegetables. Eating them raw provides the best health benefits but you can lightly cook them; keep in mind that the more you cook them, the less nutritional value they will have.

Nuts are a double-edged sword; they are good for you but they are a high calorie food item. If you are trying to lose weight or trying to maintain weight, nuts need to be eaten in moderation but the good thing is that it only takes a small serving to reap big nutritional rewards from nuts.

Nuts are packed full of fiber and protein and include minerals such as magnesium, zinc, iron and potassium. Nuts are another source of Omega-3 fatty acids and they are necessary for brain health, digestive health, skin health and for fighting off cancer causing agents in the body. There are a variety of nuts to choose from, grab a handful as a snack, mix into oatmeal or add to salads.

Avocados were once thought to be unhealthy because they have a high fat content. However, further studies have shown the avocado is full of the good type of fat, which are monosaturated fats.

A diet that included monosaturated fats can reduce bad cholesterol levels. This is not the only health benefit of avocados. Avocados contain folate, which is necessary for cardiovascular health.

Potassium helps to prevent strokes and high blood pressure. Antioxidants help keep your body healthy by attacking dangerous elements such as free radicals. Lastly, avocados contain vitamin E, which keeps the skin from aging prematurely.

Eating fresh fruit is another way to ensure that your diet is full of vitamins, antioxidants and phytonutrients, which are plant compounds that help our health. Bioflavonoids and beta-carotene are two examples of phytonutrients that are essential to good health.

Fruits and melons are excellent for keeping your body and brain healthy and working well, fighting off the signs of aging.

Nearly all berries are full of antioxidants but the blue and black berries such a blueberries, black grates, black currants and blackberries carry the biggest healthy benefit. Full of antioxidants and flavonoids, they ward off aging in the cells. Berries are also good for helping with memory function and for helping with coordination.

Starchy vegetables and colorful vegetables are also good for brain health and for providing your body with the tools that it needs to help ward off illness, disease, cancer and aging.

Beets, carrots, yams, squash, peppers (any kind or color), eggplant, radishes, and tomatoes all provide essential nutrients for your health.

Let us talk about supplements now. Taking a daily vitamin is necessary for your health, but that does not mean that you should not be eating well.

You should be doing both to ensure optimal health. Here are some of the vitamins that you need to be taking daily:

• Vitamin B12 – Lack of this vitamin causes memory problems, mood changes, and neurological problems that can include dementia and incontinence.

• Vitamin D – Vitamin D helps prevent osteoporosis, high blood pressure, heart disease, high cholesterol, diabetes and cancer. Taking vitamin D will help improve your memory and provide a mood lift.

• Vitamin C and Vitamin E – When taken together, vitamin C and vitamin E help prevent memory loss. Taking them together also lowers your risk of dementia and Alzheimer's development.

Your nutrition affects how your body ages; eat the wrong things, you age quicker; eat the right things, and you can hold off on many signs of aging as well as help keep age related illness at bay.

Exercise to Stay Young

Exercise is not only good for your health but it helps you stay young. Daily exercise helps you feel better and look better; it helps control weight, help with insomnia, control pain (especially from arthritis) and it helps prevent age related diseases such as high blood pressure, osteoporosis, cancer and heart disease.

If you want to stay younger looking and feeling, you need to get between twenty to thirty minutes of mild to moderate exercise daily.

Patients who exercise daily have longer telomeres than those who do not exercise daily. Daily exercise helps keep the telomeres from becoming shorter sooner than they should; helping keep the effects of aging at bay.

If you want to stay young, get up and get moving. Being sedentary makes you age faster, your cells will age faster if you do not exercise than if you do.

Exercise keeps your muscles from getting weak, helps keep your coordination and balance better and keeps your joints moving and lubricated.

Your muscles and joints begin to weaken as you age; joints get stiff and your natural joint lubrication can dry up, causing painful inflammation. Exercise prevents this from happening so you feel better and have less pain. Muscles that are regularly used are better able to balance so your chances of falling decrease.

Exercise also boosts your brainpower, helping to keep your brain engaged, active, and less likely to have age related problems. Exercise helps keep several areas of your brain active and fit, including the areas of your brain that handle balance, timing, decision making and learning. So to keep your brain fit, exercise your body. You benefit from it all around.

You do not have to have a gym membership or spend money on expensive and bulky equipment. As long as you are up and moving, you are getting exercise.

No matter what your fitness level is, you can find an activity that is well suited to you, as your fitness level increases then you can change your exercises accordingly. Exercising until you are a sweaty mess is also not necessary. If you are trying to lose weight, then yes, you need to work up a good sweat but for most people, even twenty minutes a day of mild exercise is good.

If you can do moderate exercise, that is better do not feel that just because you can only start off with a mild workout that it will not be good enough.

One of the problems with exercise is that it feels like work and so people give up quickly. Who wants to do something for half hour a day that they do not enjoy?

Nobody! Make your daily exercise something that you enjoy doing. If you are not having fun, it is not worth doing. Experiment with a variety of exercises so you do not get bored.

Exercise is better with a friend so enlist a friend or a group of friends to exercise with you. If you do not have anybody willing to do so, check out your community centers for free or cheap classes that you can take.

Classes are a great way to get support and help, especially if you are just getting back into being active. Being around a group of people, all supporting each other is a great way to ease back into an active lifestyle.

Try mixing up your exercise routine, walk one day, use hand weights another day, yoga another day and bike riding after that. Keep in mind that activities such as gardening count as exercise as well. If you prefer walking, change your location often so you get a change of scenery.

Not only will a change of routine keep your brain engaged, but also it will keep you from getting bored with your exercise routine. By doing a variety of activities and exercises it guarantees that you are working different muscle groups for optimal health, and not just the same muscle group over and over.

Strength training at least two to three times a week significantly cuts down on the risk of developing osteoporosis, which is a leading cause of broken bones and fractures as we age. You do not need to have heavy weights, you just need light weights to improve muscle tone and strength and keep your joints working. Use light weights to the point of feeling tired and that will be just as effective as trying to work out with heavier weights.

Walking is great exercise and you can do it anywhere. Walking is perfect for every fitness level and you can walk at a pace that suits you.

Walking is good for cardiovascular health, brain health and it helps you control your weight. Walking can be as simple as going to a local park or even just going around the block a few times.

Yoga and tai chi are two low intensity exercise methods that help boost your mental health, improve your muscle strength and your balance. Tai chi involves slow movements combined with breathing exercises and it is perfect for anybody who has not been active but wants to be.

The slow movements are great for sore joints and with daily sessions, you will start to see health benefits. Same with yoga, it is a set of specific movements along with breathing exercises that help you stay limber and gain better flexibility and balance.

Staying active means you stay young. Even though getting older comes with aches and pains, regular exercise will help minimize the pain that you can be experiencing. Your body, mind and spirit will benefit greatly by daily exercise; how and what you choose to do to be active is up to you.

Factors That Make You Older

In addition to doing things to make you look and feel younger, certain things in your life can be aging you quicker than you should be.

These factors are making you older and all of the benefits of the chapters prior to this will be cancelled out by these factors. If you want to be well and to be young, these factors need to be addressed immediately.

If you smoke, you are not doing your appearance any favors. Smoking not only carries considerable health risks to your body, but it affects your skin negatively. Chronic smoking causes the blood vessels in your skin to shrink. The blood vessels that are in your skin are already small and smoking shrinks them further.

This means that your skin is no longer getting a healthy source of blood flow. Without blood to bring nourishment to the skin, the cells become damaged.

Smoking also robs your skin of minerals and vitamins that are needed for it to stay healthy. Smoking breaks down collagen, so your skin will sag and lose its ability to be elastic. Aging dries the skin and ages it quickly, causing wrinkles and dry spots. The physical act of smoking causes wrinkles around the eyes and mouth, which will become permanent.

The diminished flow of blood in the skin means that you heal slower, so your skin scars easier. Small sores and cuts take twice as long to heal, making you look unsightly.

Smoking is one of the worst things that you can do for your skin so if you smoke and you want to look younger, you need to kick your nicotine habit. The good news is that once you stop smoking, your blood vessels will go back to normal, vastly improving the look and feel of your skin.

Chronic drinking is also very bad for your skin. Drinking on occasion is fine, but when occasionally turns into alcoholism, that is a recipe for trouble, both for your health and for your looks. Alcohol can cause a myriad of problems, none of them good.

Chronic drinking enlarges the blood vessels, especially on the face. The blood vessels around your nose and cheeks will be visible, giving your nose and face a splotchy, red appearance.

Alcohol will cause dehydration, drying out your skin, making it dry and older looking. Your kidneys will have to work harder when you drink, and this can lead to kidney problems.

If you have a daily drinking problem, seek help. Drinking does your skin no favors. If you are engaging in the occasional drink, make sure to increase your water consumption on those days to help ward off the dehydrating effects that drinking has on your body.

Illegal drugs are illegal for a reason; they will kill you. If they do not kill you, they will certainly take a serious toll on your health and your looks. Both cocaine and methamphetamine will make users look decades older than what they really are. If you have a drug habit, you need to get help and stop using right away.

If you are overweight, it takes a toll on your body, your health and your brain. Being overweight has been linked to the brain beginning to atrophy and the first part of the brain that is affected is your memory center, the hippocampus.

If you are trying to think and feel younger, being overweight does no favors to your brain. The more extra weight you carry, the more it affects your brain. If you want to ward off the negative brain effects that aging have on your brain, shed the extra weight.

Daily exercise and a good diet will help you get down to a healthy weight. Once you start to lose weight, you will look better and you will feel better. Feeling and looking better is its own motivation and you will be inspired to keep doing well with your daily exercise and diet.

There are several medical conditions that can make you feel and look older than you are. Some of these we have already gone over, such as dementia and Alzheimer's disease but the list of underlying conditions that can be aging you is large.

If you have an underlying medical condition, you need to be under the care of a doctor because leaving it untreated will age you and negatively affect your health. If you have a major medical condition, speak to your doctor about how to manage it properly.

Medication comes with its own risk. Side effects happen with all medication and the more medication you are taking, the bigger the chance of having side effects are.

Medications can cause memory loss, confusion, blurry vision or other side effects that can mimic age related diseases. It is scary to think that a great deal of the people who have been diagnosed as having dementia or Alzheimer's disease may not have the disease but their symptoms may be the result of their medication.

In addition to the above, environmental toxins also take a toll on your looks and your health. The sun is a major cause of premature aging; it causes wrinkles and dry skin.

Anytime you go out in the sun, you should be wearing sunscreen. Never spend any extending time outside without using sunscreen or sunblock because the harmful rays of the sun will age your skin and increase your risk of skin cancer.

You might think that you are doing yourself a favor by drinking diet soda but you would be wrong. The cons to drinking diet soda far outweigh the benefits of a reduced calorie drink.

Diet soda has actually been linked to an increase in belly fat in diet soda drinkers. The artificial sweeteners used in diet sodas actually cause you to store extra fat, trigger a craving for sweets and make you feel hungry. Artificial sweeteners also are linked to brain tumors, Alzheimer's and memory loss. Diet sodas should be cut from your diet right away.

Age is something that we cannot stop; but we can make some lifestyle changes to slow down the aging process and by cutting out negative habits and dangerous substances from our bodies, it helps us both look and feel younger.

It is impossible to hide from every toxic substance that will age us prematurely but the substances in this list are certainly things that we can control.

Staying Mentally Young

Mental activity and stimulation are important if you want to help keep your brain in good working order. Those who actively engage their minds are far less likely to develop Alzheimer's or dementia.

The brain has a use it or lose it aspect; if you stop using it, your mental capacity will diminish over time. Because memory problems are common with aging, keeping your brain activity will help ward off these unwelcome brain changed. If you do not want to have as many memory and brain problems as you get older, keep your brain active.

In short, the more mental activity you engage in, the more resilient your brain is towards the changes that come with age. Mental activity also reduces your risk as Alzheimer's. In order to stay young, you need to exercise more than just your body; you need to exercise your mind as well.

You do not need to sign up for formal education in order to stimulate your brain, but learning something new certainly helps! Check out local community classes for classes that might interest you.

Not only will it get your brain working, but also it gets you up and out of the house, meeting new people and having fun. Education comes in many forms and there is a variety of things that you can do to keep yourself mentally stimulated such as:

- Reading – Reading is a good way to get your mind moving. TV and movies leaves very little to the imagination. Reading engages your brain because as you read, your brain fills in the blanks for you, making the reading material come alive in your head. Spend some time every day reading, not only is it relaxing, but it is entertaining and fun. Subscribe to magazines, there are a variety of magazines that carry information that is both informative and entertaining and reading them helps engage your brain. If you always read fiction, add some non-fiction writing into your reading mix. If you only read non-fiction, add some fiction. Branching out to new genres of books helps keep your mind occupied.

- Learn a new language – Learning a new language means that you are certainly exercising your brain, helping to ward off declining mental capacity. When you learn a new language, you also help improve your overall cognitive skills so the benefits of learning a new language are easy to see. You can learn new languages at home or by taking a class.

- Take a class – There are many opportunities for learning so take advantage of them. Check with community colleges, community centers, craft stores and even museums about classes that they offer. Craft stores often have classes about new hobbies and fun skills, so you can learn and have fun at the same time. Choose a new skill, choose a new hobby or even take a cooking class; as long as you are learning something new and are having fun, it will improve your brain health.

• Teach a class – The exact opposite of taking a class is teaching a class. Share your wisdom and skills with others. You can volunteer as a class teacher or find a paid position, check around to see what opportunities are out there and help get others learning as well. This is fun and rewarding.

• Use the internet as a learning tool – There are ample learning opportunities online. Many universities offer free online lectures; you are not graded, but you can learn along. Find something that interests you and learn about it online.

• Explore different places – How many local places have you not visited? It could be parks, museums or other interesting places that you just never took the time to go see. Seeing new places and experiencing new things is great for keeping your mind stimulated. If you are able to, make a habit of traveling to new places outside of your city. Go see places that you have not seen, be a tourist and have fun.

• Be creative – When you create, you stimulate your brain. Music, art, crafting and writing are excellent for keeping your brain healthy because the creative process is very stimulating. Creativity also lowers stress levels and promotes a feeling of well-being. If you love music, but cannot play it, even just listening to music helps improve brain function. If you have never written before, start a blog; it can be fun to have a place to put down your thoughts daily.

When you do not use your brain, the neural connections begin to degrade and will die. If you want to have a healthy brain, you need to keep challenging it.

Variety is important; you cannot read the same book over and over again and continue to get the benefits of reading from it. You might enjoy the book, but it will no longer be mentally stimulating. You need to continue to find new ways to occupy your brain in order to keep your neurons from dying.

The above were ideas to help with brain health and enrich your life, but brain training focuses on keeping your brain health only.

Brain training involves doing things that require thought. Memory games, word games, crossword puzzles, search a word, and Sudoku are all popular puzzles and games that are used to help improve brain function.

There are numerous websites devoted to brain training such as Luminosity.com, RealAge.com and Prevention.com that offer brain training games online to help keep you mentally sharp. Many of the games involve engaging your memory, problem solving skills, concentration, language skills and your focus.

Do you get a daily newspaper? Most newspapers have daily puzzles in them that you can work to keep your brain sharp. If you do not get the newspaper, you can buy books of puzzles at the store to work on. Keep in mind that you only get the benefit from brain training if it is challenging so if you only work the easy puzzles, you get very little benefit from it.

Challenge yourself by working on the harder puzzles as well as the easy ones. If you normally only work crossword puzzles but not Sudoku, then start doing the Sudoku puzzles as well. Get out of your comfort zone a little bit and your brain will thank you.

The benefits of brain training include increased confidence, increased reading comprehension, better vision, quicker reaction time, improved communication skills, improved organizational skills and an increase in creativity.

Brain training is necessary to not only keep away the signs of aging in the brain but to also improve how the brain works. Daily brain training helps us think better and protects our brains from age related diseases at the same time.

You can do your own brain training daily as well, without the use of puzzles. There are a variety of things you can do daily to keep your brain active.

The idea is to challenge your brain, to make it work harder than it normally does. You can do these simple mental exercises anywhere and just doing a one of these once a day for an extended period of time will help your brain stay healthy.

Perhaps the most challenging is to switch hands. If you are eating in public, this might not be the best time to try this, especially with soup because it can be messy.

If you are used to using your dominated hand for everything, making the switch to your other hand tests your coordination and gives your brain one heck of a workout. It is hard and that is why it works, your brain has to work that much harder to work with your non-dominate hand than your dominate one.

Try doing some daily chores with your eyes closed. Take a shower with your eyes closed or try getting dressed with your eyes closed. Your brain has to work harder when you do normal tasks with your eyes closed.

It does not have to be a complicated task, even little ones, when done with your eyes closed, force your brain to use more connections, making it stronger.

Write a short story; a very short story. Write a story in ten words or less. It is harder than it sounds but very fun. When you have ten words to tell a whole story, you have to pick those words very carefully. This is a fun mental puzzle that you can do. Write one short story daily.

If you have a regular analog watch with a dial, wear it upside down. It takes a minute for you to figure out what time it is but that short amount of time where your brain is working out the time is very good for keeping your brain healthy.

Some watches run backwards or are upside down already and many people look for these types of watches rather than just putting theirs on upside down.

Conclusion

The anti-aging secret is not found in a bottle or as a cream. It is not found in a surgeon's office. The secret to anti-aging begins with you and your lifestyle. Time marches on for everybody but you hold the power for staying younger longer, both mentally and physically.

Looking younger is a big business; numerous companies target the aging demographic, promising that their products will turn back the clock if you buy their product, use their creams, or follow their fad diets. People pay a lot of money in their quest for a younger looking face and body but these products are not a full body approach.

Staying young is not just about being healthy, it is about being well. Your wellness includes your mental, physical and spiritual health. If you want to stay younger, you need to be well.

If you are fit but your mental health is not the best, you are not well. Wellness is when all three areas are in balance and that balance is what will keep you young.

Anti-aging is so much more than just how you look, it is how you act, how you think, and how healthy your body is.

Aging takes a toll on the body. Knowing how aging targets your body gives you the ammunition that you need to fight back and keep the signs of aging away. Just because you are getting older, it does not mean that you have to accept the signs of aging.

You can fight back and the information in this book will help keep you healthy and younger by taking a full wellness approach to staying young.

When you have a healthy spirit and attitude, you are a happier and healthier person. Staying positive, staying involved and staying stress free helps you stay younger and makes your life fuller and more enriching.

Being emotionally healthy helps you stay young because stress has been linked to accelerated aging by many studies.

Having a healthy body also helps you stay young. When you stay active, your joints and muscles stay healthier, helping to keep away problems with muscle tone, balance, and pain with movement.

Not only does exercise help with your health, but it keeps your body working so that it helps you feel and look younger.

Your diet impacts your health as well. If you want to feel younger and look younger, you have to give your body what it needs. So much of the average's person diet is made up of foods that are not healthy, doing us more harm than good. Skipping processed foods and going with fresh foods that are rich in antioxidants and vitamins will help you stay young and healthy.

Your brain needs exercise too and that is why learning new things and daily brain training are so important. Your brain stays active and your chance of developing dementia or Alzheimer's will be reduced.

Regular use of your brain helps improve your overall cognitive functions as well so your memory stays sharper, as does your ability to concentrate, focus and communicate. An active brain is a healthy brain.

Changes to your diet, your lifestyle and your way of thinking are necessary for the wellness approach for staying young but it works. You will look and feel younger and better than ever.